Plants inside? Why not!

This is also a cookbook

Carol J. Taylor

Contents

Chapter One

Recipe from the garden

Maintaining a patio garden is a close matter. Containers need more attention than garden parcels. Sunlight exposure is often limited, watering needs to be monitored almost daily, and efficient use of limited space can be difficult. As for myself, my patio has many pitfalls with pots and ingredients! But in the end it's worth it. Every time you harvest something from the garden and prepare a meal, you can enjoy a sweet feeling of satisfaction. It's refreshing that you don't have to rush to the store for something green. It's also great to be influenced by what's available. I don't always know what to cook, but I often find answers or at least inspiration from a quick glance at the garden. Plants thrive better when you are actively harvesting or pruning them. If harvested regularly, most plants will continue to grow and bear fruit. That's good because the kitchen is constantly supplied during the high season of summer. If you have your own garden, you learn that plants determine what you eat and vice versa. When the salad is ready, it's ready and you can enjoy the salad. Borage leaves are only a few weeks young and tender, so this is a great time to understand how to incorporate them into your diet. If you slip through the windows of these opportunities, you run the risk of becoming spoiled, bitter, or unsavory food. When thinking about gardening recipes, I follow some basic principles. I like to keep it fresh and make the flavors shine. For me, the simpler the recipe, the better. My guess is that most people don't like overly complex foods, and when you cook with herbs and flowers, you don't have to do much to emphasize their taste. I also want to use as many plants as possible. Stems, leaves, flowers, all of it. If I let something go too long and its leaves are yellowed, I use that, too. Make it your goal to leverage all the energy you`ve put into keeping the plant alive and well; you can do this by using every last bit to your advantage.  Admittedly, some of the plants in Chapter 3, What to Grow, For Real, are not familiar choices for most people. I`ve included a lot of flowers and herbs because those plants do well in containers. They may well be completely new to you, and so we get to the adventure of experimentation in the garden and the kitchen. This is a great opportunity to expand horizons and try something new. Eat something different. Challenge your palate in a new way. Make sure to pick leaves off your plants as they grow to see what they taste like. Only you know what you like!

Recipes

To Start

Zucchini Fritters

This is an easy recipe to use up a garden glut of zucchini (a wonderful container plant) and odds and ends of herbs you have growing. It`s also light and summery. Feel free to experiment with the herbs you use, but go for a mix of tender herbs (such as mint or tarragon) rather than those that prefer some cooking time (like the hardier sage and thyme). The recipe multiplies easily, so you can also adjust the quantity of this dish up given the number of guests you`re feeding. Makes 4 to 6 fritters

- 3 tablespoons olive oil, plus more for frying
- ½ onion, finely chopped (about 1 cup)
- Salt
- 2 cups finely diced zucchini (about 2 medium)
- 2 eggs
- 2 tablespoons flour, allpurpose or whole wheat
- ¼ teaspoon freshly ground black pepper

• ¼ cup chopped fresh herb mix—mint, anise hyssop, tarragon

Place a large sauté pan over medium heat, and add the olive oil. Add the onions and a pinch of salt. Sauté until the onions are soft and translucent, 8 to 10 minutes. Add the zucchini and another pinch of salt. Sauté until the zucchini is soft and nearly cooked through, another 3 minutes. Remove from the heat and spread in a single layer on a sheet pan to cool to room temperature.

In a medium bowl, whisk together the eggs, flour, pepper, and herbs. Fold the cooled zucchini mixture into the eggs until all has been incorporated. You should have a thin batter that holds together but is loose. Heat a large skillet over medium heat and cover the bottom with a thin layer of olive oil. When the pan is hot, add small ladles full of zucchini batter to form fritters about 4 inches in diameter. Fry both sides until golden. It takes about 4 to 5 minutes per side. Repeat with the rest of the dough. Eat immediately.

Other Garden Recipes: Zucchini tastes raw and is perfect for summer salads. For a simple panzanella salad, diced zucchini into small cubes, tossed with mashed tomatoes, croutons, mint and basil, and sprinkled with olive oil and red wine vinegar.

Chives butter and radish toast

This appetizer is an easy way to give guests a little treat when the time is short. Chives and radishes are one of the first vegetables available in the spring. 24 times toast

- 2 tablespoons of finely chopped chives
- 4 tablespoons of unsalted butter at room temperature
- Baguette, thinly sliced
- 1 bunch of radishes, trimmed vegetables, washed well
- Coarse sea salt

Preheat the oven to 400 ° F. Place the chives and butter in a small bowl and puree behind the spoon until well mixed. Refrigerate and set. Place a single layer of

baguette slices on a large top plate and bake for about 12 minutes until crispy and the edges begin to burn. Remove and allow to cool completely. While the crostini is cold, slice the radish using the thinnest setting of the mandolin. If you don't have a mandolin, use a knife to slice as thinly as possible to make it almost translucent. When the crostini has cooled completely, polish the top with a thin layer of chives butter. Place a slice of radish on top and layer a little. Sprinkle with sea salt and serve on a platter.

Layer crostini, chives butter, radishes and salt until the radishes are gone. Eat immediately. Wrap the remaining chives butter tightly in a wrap and store it in the freezer.

Other Garden Recipes: Chives are the ultimate accompaniment to many dishes. It has a strong onion flavor and goes very well with lean meats (grilled steaks, burgers, etc.). Chives also go well with plain boiled potatoes. Skip the butter and stir the cooked mashed potatoes with chives and salt.

Salt and Nigella Flatbread

This quick recipe can be whipped together in a hurry. These flatbreads are reminiscent of pita bread, but not nearly as doughy. They are made with whole wheat flour, which makes them dense and hardy. Nigella seeds have a slight onion taste and are beautiful seeds to use as garnish for this flatbread. • Makes 10 to 12 flatbreads

- 1½ cups whole wheat flour
- ½ cup allpurpose flour
- 1 tablespoon olive oil, plus more for brushing (or melted butter)
- Scant ¾ cup warm water
- Coarse sea salt
- 2 tablespoons nigella seeds

Combine the flours, olive oil, and water in the bowl of an electric mixer fitted with a dough hook and knead on mediumslow setting for 5 to 7 minutes, until all the flour is incorporated and the dough is elastic, not wet. Remove from the bowl, cover with a cloth, and set aside to rest for one hour. Preheat the oven to 400˚F. Set a sheet pan in the oven to heat. Cut off pieces of dough into small balls—about the size of a PingPong ball. On a lightly floured surface, roll each ball into a thin flat disk, about 5 inches across. When you have five or six disks of dough, remove the sheet pan from the oven and place the disks on the hot pan. Bake until the edges are just golden brown, 8 to 10 minutes. Continue baking the rest of the dough in this fashion. While the flatbreads are still warm, brush one side with olive oil, sprinkle with salt, and finish with a sprinkling of nigella seeds. Serve warm or hold at room temperature. Other Garden Recipes: Nigella seeds are perfect for soups and hearty vegetable dishes. Crush into a paste and go well with the plums stored with the cheese platter. Pea dumplings

In many cultures, delicious cakes and dumplings are included in the dish. My family in Croatia eats strudel-like dough stuffed with delicious stuffing like meat and onions and sweets like apples. When I was little, my aunt Janet baked ham and mozzarella french fries, as I learned from her mother-in-law in Italy. To be honest, batters that are stuffed and fried are always crushed.

Pea plants are easy to grow in containers, and you can also cut off soft tendrils from the plants for roasting while growing for peas. This recipe goes one step further and uses strong, slightly woody old grape peas. I don't usually eat it, but if you chop it into small pieces and cook it with this recipe, it will shine. These fried dumplings are the best way to use the whole plant. You can use other tough greens in this recipe-wild dandelion greens work. (If it's very bitter, use sweet vinegar such as sherry or honey to soothe the bite before adding it to the dumplings.) This is dumpling dough, isn't it?

Yeast dough so that it is soft and does not become flaky. Allow the dough to rest for at least an hour before shaping and frying. If you don't want to wait while the dough is resting, make it the night before, cover it with plastic wrap, and leave it on the counter overnight. Make 12 dumplings

- material
- 1/2 cup of all-purpose flour
- 1/2 cup whole wheat flour
- A pinch of salt
- ¼ to ½ cup of hot water
- Filling
- 2 tablespoons of olive oil
- 1/2 onion, finely chopped (about 1 cup)
- Roughly chopped ½ pound peas vine (about 4 cups)

- Just below 1/2 cup of water
- 1/4 teaspoon of ground cumin
- 1/4 teaspoon coriander
- 1/4 teaspoon smoked paprika
- Salt and freshly ground black pepper
- Vegetable oil for deep-fried foods

Place the flour and salt in a large bowl or in a bowl of an electric mixer. Gradually add water by hand until the dough is cohesive, or while running the mixer, add a small amount of water at a time until the dough is cohesive into balls. Once you have a ball of dough, knead it on a floured work surface for about 10 minutes until the dough is elastic and smooth. Cover with plastic wrap or a damp towel and let sit on the counter for at least an hour to overnight.

For stuffing, cover the bottom of a large frying pan with olive oil and heat over medium to high heat. Add half of the onions and all the pea stalks and cook with frequent stirring to prevent the pea stalks and onions from sticking together. If the pea vine deteriorates considerably,

The onions begin to soften and add water to increase the heat. When it boils, reduce the heat and cover the pot. (Because the peas tendrils are thick and woody, boil them down to soften them.)

Heat the peas tendrils for 15 to 20 minutes until the tendrils are soft and the water is almost evaporated. Remove the lid, increase the heat to dry the vegetables and onions, and evaporate the excess water. Stir well. When the pan dries and the vegetables start to stick, transfer the mixture to a large bowl. Add the remaining onions, cumin, coriander and paprika. Season with salt and pepper and let cool. For

dumplings, cut the dough into 12 pieces and roll them between the palms to make a ball. When the dough sticks, lightly sprinkle the flour on your hands. Spread a ball of dough into a small circle 4 or 5 inches in diameter on a lightly dusted work surface.

Work one round at a time and put a spoonful of pea vines in the center. Fold the dough in half. Working from the middle out, press the sides together to create a seal. (By doing this, you are pushing out any air to prevent the dumplings from breaking open while they`re frying.) You can pinch the edges with your fingers or use the back of a fork to press a design in the dough and make sure the seal holds.

Over mediumhigh heat, heat about 1 inch of vegetable oil in a deepsided sauté pan. When the oil is hot, but not smoking, slip in about four dumplings—as many as will fit without overcrowding—and fry until golden brown, 4 to 5 minutes. Flip over with a slotted spoon and fry the other side until golden brown, about another 5 minutes. Lift with a spoon with a slot and pour into a paper bag. Fry the remaining dumplings and enjoy at warm or room temperature.

Dumplings can be made a few hours in advance and fried when ready, or frozen and wrapped tightly in a plastic bag for later frying. Other Gardening Recipes: Mature peas sprouts can also be cooked as described above and used as side dishes. Skip the spices and add a handful of toasted pine nuts and lemon squeeze instead. page

Warm peas and lemon balm

Split pea is one of the best vegetables to grow on your own. Frozen peas are not like fresh peas that are sweet and crunchy, even with short bainmaries, as needed here. Blanching the peas first and then shocking them in an ice bath is a rather tedious process, but the crispy texture created by this extra step is worth it. Peas also go great with mint. You can easily use mint instead of lemon balm in this recipe, or you can use the same amount of both herbs. For 2-4 people

- Remove a pound of peas from the shell
- 1 tablespoon butter
- 1 tablespoon of finely chopped lemon balm leaves
- Salt and freshly ground black pepper

Bring a pot of salt water to a boil. Remove the peas from the shell while the water is boiling. Set up a water bath, filling a large bowl with cold water and ice. Set aside. When the peas have been hulled, drop them into the boiling water and cook until bright green and floating, 2 to 3 minutes. Drain and immediately drop them into the icewater bath, halting the cooking process. Give them a stir to make sure they are cool, then drain and set aside. In a medium skillet over medium heat, melt the butter. Add the lemon balm and stir until the leaves make a popping sound, 2 to 3 minutes. Add the peas and stir to combine. When the peas are just heated through, about 1 minute, remove from heat and season to taste with salt and pepper. Serve immediately.

More Garden Recipes: Lemon balm is a robust herb, so it`s fine to apply it sparingly. For a summer time season solar tea, integrate torn mint and lemon balm leaves, upload water, and steep withinside the solar.

Carrots with Honey and Chervil

I like to apply small carrots on this recipe, and spring is a extraordinary time to get a few. Farmers have thinned carrots from the field, and regularly you could select out up those immature carrots on the farmers` markets for cheap. Aim to buy the smallest carrots of the bunch. If you could`t discover infant carrots, sector big carrots so that you come to be with flippantly sized carrot sticks. This recipe takes benefit of blanching the carrots, so the very last texture is crisp-tender—now no longer pretty cooked, however now no longer pretty raw. Warming up butter and honey offers them a hint of sweetness that works nicely with the taste of the chervil. You can replacement parsley for chervil in case you leave out the season—chervil is to be had in early spring and every so often in July after it reseeds itself.

Serves four to 6

- 1 pound small carrots, peeled
- 1 tablespoon butter
- 1 teaspoon honey
- 1 tablespoon more or less chopped clean chervil
- Salt and freshly floor black pepper
- Set up an ice-water bath—integrate bloodless water and a handful of ice in a big bowl.

Bring a pot of salted water to boil. Add the carrots and blanch till simply tender, approximately four minutes. Strain and right now plunge the carrots into the ice-water bath. Stir every so often till cool. Drain and set aside.

In a medium sauté pan, soften the butter over medium-excessive warmth. Stir withinside the honey. Add the carrots and prepare dinner dinner till simply warmed through, stirring continuously. Remove from the warmth and stir withinside the chervil. Season to flavor with salt and pepper. Serve right now.

More Garden Recipes: Chervil is a extraordinary healthy for eggs—scrambled, hard-boiled, you call it. Chervil additionally makes a adorable garnish for easy broth soups. For an clean and mild meal, warmth up a few hen inventory till hot, pour in a whisked egg, and prepare dinner dinner till the egg bureaucracy ribbons withinside the soup, approximately 2 minutes. Garnish with chervil.

Crispy Marjoram Potatoes

This is one in all my favourite methods to prepare dinner dinner potatoes. The trick is to position the potatoes reduce aspect down in a sauté pan over medium warmth (now no longer warmer or they`ll burn!) and depart them be. No touching! The potatoes come to be golden brown and crispy however continue to be fluffy and candy inner like a mashed potato. Potatoes and marjoram are a extraordinary healthy. For this recipe, I prepare dinner dinner 1/2 of the marjoram with the potatoes and upload 1/2 of to the completed dish for additonal herby taste. You can double up this batch to serve a crowd, however ensure you maintain the potatoes in a unmarried layer withinside the pan. You may also want to apply pans to house them all.

Serves 4

- 2 tablespoons olive oil
- 1 tablespoon butter
- 1 pound Yukon Gold or fingerling potatoes, sliced in 1/2 of lengthwise
- Salt and freshly floor black pepper
- 2 tablespoons chopped sparkling marjoram, divided

Preheat the oven to 350˚F. In a huge ovenproof sauté pan over medium warmth, warmth the olive oil and butter. When the butter is melted and hot, area potatoes into the pan in a unmarried layer, reduce aspect down. Sprinkle with a few salt and prepare dinner dinner till a pointy knife nearly pierces the center, eight to ten minutes. The potatoes will nevertheless deliver resistance and be uncooked withinside the middle. Sprinkle 1 tablespoon of the marjoram over the potatoes and area the whole pan withinside the oven.

Bake till a pointy knife without problems pierces thru the flesh, 10 to fifteen minutes. Remove from the oven and switch to a shallow serving bowl. Toss withinside the ultimate marjoram and stir to integrate. Season to flavor with salt and pepper and serve.

More Garden Recipes: Marjoram is a herbal herb for any Italian dish. For a brief tomato sauce, sauté garlic in olive oil, upload a can or jar of stewed tomatoes, and end it with some tablespoons of marjoram. Marjoram additionally tastes outstanding with chicken; attempt substituting marjoram withinside the Thyme-Roasted Chicken Legs with Charred Onions recipe.

Smoky Chickpeas with Greens

Miner`s lettuce is a succulent inexperienced that grows wild however may be cultivated in a lawn. It is one of the first vegetables to pop up in past due iciness or early spring, so it's miles ideal for a lawn salad after months of no sparkling vegetables. Miner`s lettuce has smooth, lily-pad-like leaves and organization crisp stems. Their vegetables will preserve their shape, even after the addition of an acid, making them an outstanding addition to legume salads. In this recipe, the acid from a lemon cuts the chew from the uncooked onion. The addition of chickpeas makes for a mild lunch. This is an smooth recipe to multiply for guests.

Serves 1

- three skinny slices pink onion
- ½ lemon, zested and juiced
- three tablespoons olive oil

- ¼ teaspoon smoked paprika
- ¼ teaspoon salt
- ½ cup chickpeas, cooked
- 1 cup miner`s lettuce or different spring lettuces
- Salt and freshly floor black pepper

In huge bowl, integrate the onion and lemon juice. Let stand for five to ten minutes. Then upload the lemon zest, olive oil, paprika, salt, and chickpeas. Stir properly and permit take a seat down for at the least 15 minutes. Toss withinside the miner`s lettuce and stir to blend. Season to flavor with salt and pepper and serve immediately.

More Garden Recipes: Miner`s lettuce is going properly with different early and hardy vegetables like arugula. Make a easy salad the use of each vegetables and something herbs you've got got around. Miner`s lettuce is likewise a first rate alternative for watercress in recipes. Try including a few leaves to a creamy potato soup and blending.

Pickled cucumber and sesame toast salad

I always make this salad, and my friends always ask me for a "recipe". They are usually shocked to know how little material they have. "Is that it?" Everyone asks incredibly. Basically, soak the cucumbers in sake vinegar quickly. Additional hints for toasted flavors come from both sesame oil and toasted sesame seeds. If you don't have a seed at hand, you can easily skip the seed. Serves 2 to 4

- 3 tablespoons rice wine vinegar
- 2 teaspoons sugar
- 1 pound cucumbers, peeled and sliced thin
- 1 teaspoon sesame oil
- 1 teaspoon sesame seeds, toasted

In a shallow bowl, combine the vinegar and sugar. Add the cucumbers and toss to coat. Set aside to macerate for 30 minutes or so, stirring often to rotate the cucumber slices. After 30 minutes, add the sesame oil and toasted sesame seeds. Stir to combine and serve. Other garden recipes: Finely chop cucumbers and combine with tarragon for a summer treat of grilled fish. Alternatively, chop the cucumber into small pieces and mix with natural yogurt to make zucchini fritters. Cucumbers go well with melons in fresh salads and raw soups.

mint rocket salad

Arugula and mint are in perfect harmony. One leaf is spicy and the other is chilled. This salad can be finely chopped and used as a side dish for sliced tomatoes or grilled meat. You can mix the two in pesto to marinated fish or toss pasta. (Both variations require a little more olive oil than listed here.) Another option is to leave whole leafy vegetables, as we did here for side salads. Feel free to play with proportions. The salad should be light. I rarely measure the ingredients. I plan only a handful of vegetables per person. For 2 people as a small salad

- 1 cup arugula
- ¼ cup of mint leaves, torn
- 2 tablespoons of olive oil
- ½ lemon, grated, juice
- Salt and freshly ground black pepper

In a large mixing bowl, mix the arugula, mint, olive oil, lemon juice and rind. Adjust the taste with salt and pepper. Eat immediately.

Other Garden Recipes: Arugula is the perfect green to add flavor and texture to your salad. If your plant goes to flower, pick off small.

Leaves and use the white flower heads in salads. Because its taste is so strong, you may additionally contain arugula into soups. Make a white bean soup and upload a handful or of arugula whilst you combination it smooth. It provides a pleasing highly spiced note.

Roasted Shiitakes with Fennel Blossoms

Roasted mushrooms are an smooth and flavorful facet dish any time of the yr. Shiitakes are broadly cultivated and to be had all yr long. They don`t have an awful lot moisture, in order that they bake as much as a chewy-crisp texture quickly. For this recipe, mushrooms are roasted till the stems simply start to brown. Fennel blossoms may be accrued in summer time season and stored as a spice withinside the pantry. They impart a candy fennel taste and aroma to those mushrooms this is pretty distinct, in addition to phenomenally flavorful.

Serves four

- 2 kilos shiitake mushrooms, kind of torn into pieces
- 1 teaspoon salt
- ½ teaspoon freshly floor black pepper
- 1 tablespoon fennel blossoms
- three tablespoons olive oil

Preheat the oven to 400˚F. Toss the mushrooms, salt, pepper, fennel blossoms, and oil in a big bowl, coating the mushrooms evenly. Spread out on a sheet pan, in a unmarried layer, and bake for 30 to forty minutes, tossing occasionally, till the mushrooms are contracted and their stems are beginning to crisp. They may have launched maximum in their moisture and reduced in size in size. Serve right away or preserve at room temperature till serving.

More Garden Recipes: Fennel blossoms are a extremely good herb to feature to red meat or a white fish like halibut. A mild sprinkle of blossoms may also upload a complementary taste to vegetable soups.

Main Dishes

Herby Pasta with Lettuce and Prosciutto

This recipe turned into one of these glad injuries I made one day. I didn`t have an awful lot withinside the pantry, and I commenced simply throwing components right into a pan. I left onions and prosciutto to take a seat down and get crispy, then doused them with a few pasta water to make a thick broth. At the closing minute, I delivered handfuls of lettuce to the pot—a extremely good manner to contain vegetables right into a pasta dish. Use something vegetables you've got got on hand—Bibb lettuce, romaine, radicchio, arugula, parsley, mint, basil, lovage, and so on. This is likewise a extremely good manner to expend any lettuce that can be beginning to bolt and flip sour or has started to wilt with age. Choose a formed pasta (bowtie is my favorite), now no longer a protracted noodle.

Serves four

- three tablespoons olive oil
- 1 tablespoon butter

- five garlic cloves, peeled and sliced
- 1 shallot
- four slices prosciutto, torn into pieces
- 1 tablespoon dry vermouth
- four cups bowtie or different formed pasta
- four cups combined lettuce vegetables
- ½ cup combined herbs
- Parmesan for garnish (optional)
- Boil a pot of salted water for the pasta.

In a large high-side frying pan, heat olive oil and butter over medium to high heat. When the butter melts and begins to foam, add garlic and shallot. Bake for about 8-10 minutes until cooked and the edges start to burn. Add prosciutto and leave for about 4 minutes, then stir occasionally to make it brown and crispy. When the mixture begins to stick to the bottom of the pan, remove the glaze with vermouth and scrape off the brown pieces. Boil the vermouth for 1 minute, then remove the pan from the heat. Put the noodles in boiling water and simmer in al dente for about 10 minutes. Bring the sauté pan back to high heat 1 minute before the noodles are complete. It begins to burn almost immediately. Pour the pasta water into the sauté pan, stirring constantly. When the pasta becomes al dente, drain it and add it to the pan. Cook for about 3 minutes until the pasta water begins to evaporate and foams at the bottom of the pan. Add a handful of vegetables and herbs at a time, toss and mash. Continue adding until it is installed and immediately remove it from the heat. Spoon 4 equal parts into a shallow bowl. If necessary, grate the Parmesan cheese on top and serve immediately. Other Gardening Recipes: Of course, homemade salads are great salads. Season with olive oil, lemon juice, salt and freshly ground black pepper. Lettuce can also be used to make salad soups. Fry the onions until cooked, add the lettuce, and add the soup and puree with a small amount of cream.

Peas falafel

Falafel is traditionally made from pure chickpeas. This version also uses peas. I learned from my friend Mark, the chef and owner of Spring Hill, a popular Seattle restaurant. We leveled Mark's backyard many years ago and since then I've been growing produce for restaurants. Recently he and I gave a cooking demonstration-he cooked, I talked about how to grow food. He took the excess of peas from the garden and made a flavorful fried falafel. weather. It's also a healthy dish. Try falafel wrapped in salty Nigella flatbread (page 83) with pickles and a spoonful of yogurt. Served 4

- 1¼ cup chickpeas

• 1¼ cup peas with shells

• 1/2 large onion, chopped

• Chickpea flour ¼ cup

• 1/2 teaspoon baking soda

• 1 teaspoon of salt

• 1 teaspoon of smoked paprika

• 1 teaspoon curry powder

• 1 teaspoon of Garam masala

• 1/4 teaspoon freshly ground black pepper

• 1/4 teaspoon cayenne pepper

• 1 cup of fresh herbs such as lemon balm, mint, anise, hyssop, lavage, tarragon, parsley and coriander

• ½ lemon, grated, juice

• Olive oil for deep-fried food

The night before, soak the chickpeas in a bowl of cold water on the counter chickpeas. Drain well in the morning, and if it's still damp, tap it to dry. Bring a pot of salt water to a boil. Set up a water bath and fill a large bowl with cold water and ice. Set aside. Add the peas removed from the shell to boiling water and heat for 2-3 minutes until they float in a light green color. If you drain it and immediately drop it in an ice bath, the cooking process will stop. Stir to make sure they are cold, then drain and set aside. Place chickpeas and peas in a bowl of steel blade food processor. Add all other materials. Disassemble and mix until well mixed. The dough is almost pasty and should be held together. If it's too damp, add a spoonful of chickpea flour. Scrape it from the processing bowl into another bowl and leave it for 30 minutes. In a large frying pan, add enough olive oil to cover the bottom of the pan and lift the sides slightly. Heat on medium heat. in the case of

The oil is hot, so add a spoonful of falafel batter and fry. Do not move the falafel as the batter will be quite soft. Wait for one side to have a nice golden color before turning it over. Continue to fry on all sides until golden. Remove from the pan and drain on a paper bag. Repeat with the remaining batter. Serve immediately.

EDIBLE BLOSSOMS

Many plants produce flowers that are edible, often with a more muted version of the plant`s leaf, stem, or root flavor. These blossoms can be harvested and eaten as well! They make a pretty presentation, and it`s a good way to use all of the plant before pruning after bloom. Anise hyssop: Soft licorice flavor. Flower heads form many individual flower spikes. To harvest, close the fists around the buds and pull down the stems to remove the buds.

Scented geranium: Tastes just like the plant variety`s specific heady fragrance and is tremendous candied for garnish.

Squash: These massive orange plants don`t flavor like an awful lot, however their length makes them best for stuffing and cooking. Make positive you harvest handiest male blossoms (with a stamen—believe me, it ought to be obvious) and depart the lady blossoms to provide fruit.

Thyme: Tiny little plants which are strongly flavored like thyme.

More Garden Recipes: Peas make a amazing filling; you may mash them to fill ravioli or savory tarts. Try changing 1/2 of of the ricotta withinside the filling for the Borage Zucchini Tart (web page 101) with mashed peas. Whole peas also are tremendous served with lengthy pasta noodles. Make a brief sauce with prosciutto and butter in a sauté pan, upload the peas, then toss with pasta. Finish with clean mint and a grate or of lemon zest.

Seared Pork Chops and Fennel Blossoms with Fig-Lovage Relish

I love figs, and I actually have lengthy been keen on lovage, which merits to be an awful lot extra extensively known. Lovage tastes like a more potent model of a celery leaf. As its taste is extra pronounced—a bit is going an extended way. I serve this get pleasure from with seared red meat chops, however it'd be amazing on maximum roasted meats or a fatty fish like black cod. The red meat chops are gently rubbed with fennel blossoms (which may be harvested from the wild in summer), beaten coriander seeds, and paprika. It`s a pleasing smoky aggregate of flavors to play off the beauty of the figs. Feel loose to leave out the rub absolutely and really season the red meat with salt and pepper; it'll be similarly delicious.

Relish

To make the get pleasure from, chop the figs into small dice. Add the lovage, sherry vinegar, and olive oil to the figs. Stir and set apart to macerate.

To make the rub, integrate the fennel blossoms, coriander, salt, and pepper. Sprinkle the rub on each aspects of every of the chops, and pat it in. You need a quite skinny sprinkling, now no longer a thick layer, so use sparingly, however use it all.

To make the red meat chops, warmness the olive oil and butter in a massive sauté pan over medium warmness. When the butter is melted and effervescent at the rims and the pan is hot, upload the red meat chops. Let sear till golden brown. Don`t flow the chops around, simply allow them to take a seat down and color. After approximately 6 minutes, you may see that the edges of the chops are starting to prepare dinner dinner. Flip them over and prepare dinner dinner till cooked via and firm, some other five to six minutes. Remove the chops to a plate and allow them to rest. Return the pan to the stovetop and growth the warmth to high. The brown bits withinside the pan will begin to sizzle and burn. Splash withinside the vermouth and quick scrape free all of the bits. Cook for 1 minute extra, then dispose of from warmness.

To serve, place one pork chop per person on a plate and decorate with a spoonful of relish. Spread the gravy evenly on the chops and serve immediately. Other garden recipes: Lovage is a natural accompaniment to shellfish. Steam a large pot of lajonkairia or mussels and add lavage when adding shellfish. Lovage goes great with eggs. For a healthy breakfast, softly boil the eggs, puree the toast, and add chopped lavage leaves and salt. Roast chicken drumstick with thyme and roasted onions

When roasting chicken, the first thing to grab is inevitably the thigh. We often miss something when we let our guests choose politely and first. My friend Michelle solves this conundrum for her family by buying an additional pack of drumsticks every time she roasts chicken. Great! In this recipe, plenty of thyme is added to both chicken and onions, but the beauty really lies in roasting. Chicken starts at a very high temperature. After 20 minutes, the legs are slowly cooked at low temperature for almost an hour and come out of the oven like a "confit". The outside is crispy and the inside is juicy. The result is a simple yet soothing dish of sweet onions and crispy chicken. Thyme is a tough herb, so you can use it from the garden to winter. Served 4

- 8 chicken thighs
- salt
- 2 onions, peel and cut into medium-thick crescents or rings
- 3 tablespoons of olive oil
- 6 tablespoons chopped thyme, split and even garnish
- 1/2 teaspoon of freshly ground black pepper
- 1 lemon, grated

Prepare chicken thighs with plenty of salt at least 1 hour and 1 day before cooking. Store in a resealable plastic bag or wrap and refrigerate until ready for use. Preheat the oven to 450 ° F. In a large bowl, combine onions, olive oil and 3 tablespoons of thyme and coat with toss. Spread the onions evenly on a large top plate. In the same bowl, mix the remaining thyme, 1 teaspoon salt, pepper, lemon zest and chicken thighs. Turn it over, spice it under the skin on your feet and rub it. Place your feet directly on the onions to prevent them from touching or overlapping.

Place the sheet pan withinside the oven and roast for 20 mins. Without beginning the oven door, lessen the warmth to 350˚F and bake for forty five mins to at least one hour, till the legs are golden brown and wrinkled. Check the pan each 15 mins; if the onions alongside the rims are turning too black, toss as needed.

Remove the pan from the oven and switch the onions to a big platter. Set the legs on pinnacle of the onions and garnish with a pinch of clean thyme if desired. Serve immediately.

More Garden Recipes: Thyme is a extraordinary accomplice to lemon. Steep a spray of thyme in lemonade or make a warm tea of thyme and lemon slices with honey. You also can make simply the onions from this dish and bake them on a rectangular of puff pastry for a fast celebration appetizer. Thyme infuses well; strive substituting thyme for the anise hyssop withinside the Anise Hyssop Ice Cream (web page 108) and serve with a bowl of berries.

Borage Zucchini Tart

This tart is made in stages, however it`s really well worth the greater time. Using store-offered puff pastry, the tart is layered with borage-scented ricotta cheese and sautéed zucchini, then crowned with a lattice of zucchini slices. Laticework takes time, so in case you opt for now no longer to fuss with it, without a doubt layer zucchini in a row throughout the tart. Borage has a totally wonderful cucumberlike taste and pairs properly with zucchini. It`s a extraordinary manner to utilize a prolific box plant. If you're so inclined, you could make simply the borage-ricotta combination and serve a huge spoonful over a few pasta wearing olive oil. The cheese will also be used on crostini as an appetizer or as filling in home made ravioli. The tart may be made an afternoon ahead, wrapped loosely in parchment paper and refrigerated till equipped to serve.

Serves 4

- Flour, for dusting
- 1 sheet puff pastry
- 2 big zucchini
- 1 tablespoon butter
- 1 tablespoon olive oil
- ½ onion, finely chopped
- Salt
- 1 cup ricotta
- 30 borage leaves, chopped fine
- 1 lemon, zested
- 2 tablespoons grated Parmesan
- ½ teaspoon freshly floor black pepper
- 1 egg yolk, beaten

To prepare the pastry shells, lightly sprinkle the countertop with flour and spread the puff pastry to half its original thickness (a square of approximately 11 x 11 inches). Make a 1/4 inch wide tri-fold along both sides of the dough and fold towards the center of the dough to form the wall of the puff pastry. There is a padding on this wall. Pinch the corners firmly. Don't worry if the pastry isn't a perfect square. The dough swells as it burns and those small imperfections do not appear. Place the cake base in a can and freeze until ready for use. For iron plates, slice the zucchini vertically in the thinnest step of the mandolin, or use a knife to cut it into very thin strips vertically. Place the strips in a cooling rack set on the sheet pan and lightly salt. This helps remove some of the water from the zucchini. While the zucchini strips are being drained, cut the remaining zucchini into small, uniform cubes. Heat butter and olive oil in a large frying pan over medium to high heat. When the butter has melted, add the onions and simmer for about 8-10 minutes until soft and translucent. Add diced zucchini and a little salt and fry for about 4 minutes until the zucchini is completely cooked. Remove from heat, spread in a thin layer on the top plate and let cool. In a small bowl, mix ricotta cheese, borage, lemon zest, parmesan cheese and pepper. Press the zucchini strip between the layers of kitchen towel or paper towel to remove excess water. Preheat the oven to 375 ° F. To assemble the cake, remove the pastry shells from the freezer. Spread the ricotta cheese on the bottom of the bowl.

Spread the zucchini and onion saute evenly over the ricotta cheese. Place a slice of zucchini on top of the pie, from top to bottom, with a few layers. Work vertically on this layer and place the zucchini slices from left to right. Lift every other row of zucchini from top to bottom and insert new horizontal slices up and down to create a grid pattern. Weave the strips over the cake and push or trim the edges to prevent it from hanging on the wall of the cake. Once you have a grid, polish the entire top of the cake with egg yolk. Bake for 40-45 minutes until swelling and golden. Consume warm or at room temperature. Other Gardening Recipes: Borage flowers make a nice decoration for cocktails and summer drinks. Young borage leaves can be torn and added to the salad, adding a soft cucumber flavor. For a light summer salad, chop the borage leaves and mix with steamed shrimp, lemon juice and avocado.

Take the frozen pastry shell out of the freezer and use it to create the tart. Using the bottom of the shell, spread the ricotta. Spread the ricotta in an even layer and then top with the sautéed zucchini and onion mixture. Overlap the zucchini slices slightly as you spread them around the tart, from top to bottom. Layer zucchini slices from left to right, working in the opposite direction of this layer. Lift every other row of zucchini from top to bottom and tuck the new horizontal slices over and under to create a latticework pattern. Tuck or cut the strips' edges into the tart so they don't droop over the sides, then weave them in a pattern across the entire tart.

A brushing with egg yolk should be done after completing the lattice. Bake for 40 to 45 minutes, or until puffed and golden brown. Serve at room temperature or heated.

More Garden Recipes: Borage blossoms make a wonderful garnish for cocktails and summertime drinks. The soft cucumber flavour of young borage leaves can be added to salads by chopping them up and sprinkling them on top. Slicing the leaves of borage and tossing them with cooked shrimp, lemon juice, and avocado is a light summer salad.

Chapter Two

Dandelion Greens and Lemon Trout

As frightening as it may be to cook a whole fish for the first time, trout is one of the easiest to prepare. Commercial trout is already scaled and gutted, so there's no need to do any cleaning. It's been years since I first tried my buddy Jaime's delicious and nutritious recipe, but it's remained a go-to for me ever since. The dandelion greens and almond salad is served on top of a rapid broiler-cooked whole fish. Dandelion greens have a strong flavour, but they complement the delicate fish. Aside from being delicious, they're loaded with nutrients like vitamin A, iron, and calcium. Spring is the best time to harvest dandelion greens because the older, larger leaves are woody and bitter.

Servings Per Container: 2

1 peeled and mashed clove of garlic

almond slices, about 1 cup

• 2 handfuls of finely chopped dandelion greens

Zest and thinly slice 1 lemon.

At least one tablespoon of olive oil is required.

• Black pepper, salt, and peppercorns.

There is a single entire trout.

The broiler should be preheated and the oven rack should be moved to the highest position.

The garlic clove should be minced and ground in a mortar and pestle. Garlic should be thrown away once it has been doused in oil and has cooled. Add the almonds to the food processor and process until they are finely ground. Mash all the ingredients together with a fork until they're smooth and creamy. In terms of appearance, the mixture will be somewhere in between a salad and a pesto. The leafy portions should vary in size, but that's a good thing. Give it one last swirl with the pestle before adding the olive oil and salt. Set away for later.

Meanwhile, salt and pepper the trout on both the outside and the inside. Using a pair of scissors, cut several lemon slices into the trout's belly. To keep the trout from sticking to the pan, pour a little olive oil over them before placing them there. A sheet pan should be placed directly under a preheated broiler and blasted for 4 to 5 minutes on one side until the skin begins to shrivel and burn. The trout is done when you can easily flip it with a spatula. To finish cooking, broil the opposite side for 4 to 5 minutes until browned and cooked through.

Serve the dandelion salad alongside the grilled trout. Serve right away.

Garden Recipes: Dandelions are a nice green to add to your salad, but use them sparingly so that the other flavours don't overwhelm. Crush garlic and pine nuts into a dandelion pesto and serve it with pasta. Pea Vine Dumplings can also be filled with dandelion greens (page 84).

Chapter Three

Rice Krispies Treats with Chamomile and Coconut

Lynda, one of my closest friends, works in a goat dairy as a cheese maker. I had the pleasure of spending a few days with her in farm country last summer, and every morning for breakfast I had a large bowl of her excellent goat milk yoghurt topped with spoonfuls of her homemade granola and a generous drizzle of honey. The coconut, oats, and almonds in her granola are toasted and flaky because she doesn't use any butter or sugar in the recipe. Some chamomile buds and sesame seeds enhance the flavour. You'll never think of granola the same way again after trying this.

Serves six people.

- 1 cup oats rolled

Almonds, roughly chopped, 1 cup

• 1 cup of coconut flakes, raw and unsweetened

Salt, about a quarter-teaspoon

• 1 tbsp. of ground chamomile.

sesame seeds, untoasted, 1 Tbsp.

1 tbsp. ground flaxseed

The oven should be preheated to 350 degrees Fahrenheit before you begin baking. Stir up all ingredients in a sheet pan. Toast for 5 minutes in the oven. Take out the pan and toss it to redistribute the granola evenly. Add the coconut flakes and continue toasting for an additional 3-4 minutes, or until golden. Toss in a cup of plain yoghurt with a drizzle of honey and some fresh berries. Granola that has cooled and is in a sealed container can be stored in the pantry for up to three weeks.

Oats and chamomile are a match made in heaven. Get creative and experiment with a variety of different ways to incorporate the buds into your diet.

Chapter Four

Buttermilk Cake topped with fresh rosy strawberries

Flowers like rose geranium, which can be grown easily, work well in sweet dishes and sweets. When paired with strawberries, its floral aroma is particularly appealing. Ripe berries are macerated with sugar and chopped rose geranium leaves in this simple dish. This simple buttermilk cake is a great accompaniment to any meal. A spoonful of vanilla ice cream or the sweet rosy sauce by itself, perhaps with a squirt of cream on top, is a delicious way to enjoy this sauce.

Serves four

- Strawberries

Strawberry puree, 1 pint, smashed and quartered

16 ounces of honey

Rose geranium leaves finely cut • 5 big leaves

• Cake

• 1 cup pastry flour made from whole wheat

• 1 pound of ground beef

Baking powder, 1 tea spoon

• 1 teaspoon of baking soda

salt, about a half tsp.

• 1 quart of sour cream

The vanilla extract, 1 teaspoon

• 1 stick of room-temperature butter

• 1 cup of sugar

Eggs, two big

Sugar, finely ground (optional)

In a small bowl, combine the strawberries, sugar, and rose geranium leaves; set aside for 30 minutes before serving..

The oven should be preheated to 350 degrees Fahrenheit before you begin baking. Grease and set aside a 9-inch cake pan. Discard all except one of the dry ingredients and combine them in a small bowl. In a separate bowl, combine the buttermilk and vanilla extract; place this mixture in the refrigerator until needed.

Cream the butter and sugar with a stand mixer until fluffy, about 5 minutes. The final product should be light and fluffy. Mix in the eggs one at a time, scraping down the sides of the bowl after each addition to ensure complete incorporation. Continue to whisk until just mixed after adding one-half of the flour mixture. Once you've added the buttermilk mixture, mix it in thoroughly with a spoon. Just before serving, toss in the rest of the flour mixture. Using a toothpick placed into the middle of the cake comes out clean, bake the cake for 30 to 40 minutes.

Cool the cake on a cooling rack and dust with powdered sugar, if desired. Serve with a big dollop of berries that have been macerated in sugar.

Using rose geranium as a flavouring for ice cream or whipped cream is a simple way to get the plant into your diet without having to buy it. Try making a smoothie out of leaves, milk, and strawberries for breakfast.

The Ice Cream of Anise Hy-Sop

The conical structure of the purple anise hyssop flower at a farmers' market a few years ago sparked my interest in this plant. I couldn't help but fall in love with the flavour all over again as soon as I took a bite. The new herb, which tastes like licorice and mint, had me stumped, so I used it to flavour some ice cream. One of my favourites, I often make this with berries and cakes instead of vanilla and serve it as a side dish.

It yields around 2 pints of liquid.

12-cups-of-complete-milk

• 12 a cup of white sugar

ten leaves of anise hyssop

Egg whites and three yolks, plus one whole egg

• 112 quarts of heavy cream •

Pour the milk, sugar, and anise hyssop leaves into a medium saucepan and bring to a boil over medium heat. Allow it steep for around 30 minutes, or until you're satisfied with the flavour. Reheat the mixture over a medium-low heat.

Whisk the yolks and whites of the eggs until they are completely mixed in a glass basin. Whisk the eggs continuously as you add a ladleful of the warm milk mixture. Add another ladleful and stir until the mixture is completely smooth. In order to avoid overcooking the eggs when you add them to the saucepan, you are carefully tempering the eggs with a warm liquid.

Pour the egg mixture into the milk mixture and cook over medium heat for about 8 minutes, stirring constantly. Make sure you don't overheat. Cook until the custard is just thick enough to coat the back of a wooden spoon, constantly stirring. When you're done cooking, drain the custard into a large mixing dish to cool completely. (The anise hyssop leaves will also be removed by straining.) Stir in the heavy cream and mix until smooth. Afterwards, serve.

Refrigerate the custard for at least 4 hours or overnight, covered with plastic wrap. Cream and freeze in an ice cream maker as directed by the manufacturer, using a spatula to scrape down the sides of the basin as needed. Keep the ice cream in the freezer until ready to serve in an airtight container.

Anise hyssop leaves provide a flavorful addition to a grain or legume salad, for example. Herbal sun teas with anise hyssop are also delicious.

Chapter Five

Petals made of sugar

Despite the fact that some edible flowers are palatable, I've found that most petals don't taste like anything. When I have a flowering plant, I make sugared petals and use them as garnishes on desserts or fruit platters. Herb leaves can be used in the same way. It's not just about the taste when it comes to these tasty finishing touches; they're also about the aesthetic appeal, too.

When it comes to sugaring petals and leaves, it's a simple but time-consuming process. Clear a path for yourself. Get a cooling rack and a large dish ready for your food. Once the petals have been sugared, the cooling rack will be used to dry them. The sheet pan will catch all of the sugar that falls on it. Tweezers are a must-have as well.

To separate the petals, cut the stems from the plant and delicately dissect the head of the flower. Beat one egg white in a small bowl and thin with a few drops of water. With the help of the tweezers, pick up each petal (so your fingers don't get stuck). Apply a thin layer of egg wash to each petal with a pastry brush or small paintbrush. Brushing huge leaves is easier if you place them in the palm of your hand. Coat both sides completely. And no, you can't merely dip the leaf or petal in water—the covering is too thick.) Using tweezers, hold the leaf or petal over the sheet pan and sprinkle sugar on both sides after brushing both sides with the egg white wash. Allow to air dry on a cooling rack.

Listed below are a few gorgeous blossoms and tasty leaves that can be candied:

A hyssop leaf with an anise flavour

- Lemon verbena sprigs
- Mint sprigs are also available.
- Nasturtium
- Geranium

Chapter Six

Lavender-Chocolate Tart

A very small slice of this deep, creamy tart is all you need. Making this dessert for a dinner party is a terrific idea because it feeds anywhere from 12 to 20 people. When chocolate and milk are melted together, the result is a basic ganache. If you want a delicate or bold flavour, you can control how long the cream is infused with lavender buds. The lavender taste really shines through, so I steep the flowers for around 40 minutes in the cream. This is a recipe that needs to be made in stages, so you'll need to bake the tart shell a day in advance. At room temperature or in the fridge, this chocolate dessert can be stored for several days without deteriorating.

12 to 20 people can be fed at a time with this dish.

On the other hand, the Tart Shell

- 1 pound of ground beef

- 1 cup pastry flour made from whole wheat

salt, about a teaspoonful

- 1 tsp. of sugar

Unsalted butter, 12 pound (2 sticks), cooled, cubed

A cup of icy water with 8 teaspoons of ice

- Filling

- 1 quart of sour cream

Lavender buds, about 112 teaspoons

Finely chopped 10 ounces of dark chocolate

A total of three egg yolks

Once or twice in the bowl of a food processor fitted with a steel blade, combine the flours, salt, and sugar for the tart shell. Be cautious not to overprocess the dough when you add the butter and pulse until large crumbs form.

Dough should come together in two or three large chunks when the mixer is running and the ice water has been added slowly, 1 tablespoon at a time. It's possible that you won't need all of that water. To avoid overprocessing, it takes roughly 8 to 10 seconds.

Make two 6-inch-diameter discs by dividing the dough in half and pressing each half into a flat round disc. Avoid overworking the dough. Refrigerate for at least 2 hours after each item has been wrapped snugly in plastic wrap.

Removing the chilled dough from the fridge is the final step before using it. A work surface should be lightly dusted with flour. Roll the dough into a 10-inch circle with a rolling pin (be sure to rotate the dough and flip it over, rolling both sides). Keep the work surface lightly floured to prevent the dough from sticking.

In a detachable bottom 9-inch tart pan, insert the round and fold it in half (with the folded edge running down the middle of the pan). Disk over the side of the tart pan, folded in half. Avoid stretching it out of shape by gently pressing it into the tart pan. Apply pressure to any crust that is hanging over the sides of the pan. Make sure the top of the shell is even by running a rolling pin over it and pressing down. The bottom of the tart shell should be punctured numerous times with a fork. Before baking, put the food in the freezer for 30 minutes.

The oven should be preheated to 350 degrees Fahrenheit before you begin baking. Place the tart pan in the freezer and line the inside with parchment paper before baking. Add weights to the parchment paper in the corners with pie weights or beans.

Bake for 30 minutes on the centre rack. Continue baking for another 10 to 15 minutes after removing the pie weights and parchment. The tart shell should be taken out of the oven, cooled, and put away until use.

Mix the lavender and cream in a medium saucepan and bring to a boil over medium heat. Set it aside to infuse when it's warm. reheat if the cream gets too cold

again and let it soak for a while longer. From 20 to 40 minutes, depending on how strong a taste you want, the lavender should be steeped in the warm cream with the lavender buds.

The chocolate can be found in a separate bowl. Whisk the egg yolks in a separate bowl until they are completely incorporated.

Squeeze out any remaining bud fragments and return the cream to medium-low heat. Heat for about 2 minutes, or until it barely starts to steam. Add a few spoonfuls of cream at a time to the eggs, whisking constantly. In order to prevent the eggs from curdling due to overcooking, use this method to temper them. When you've added all of the cream to the eggs, keep whisking. Once all the cream is added and properly combined with the yolks, lay a strainer over the dish of chocolate and pour in the hot cream and egg yolk combination.

Fold the heated cream around the chocolate chunks with a rubber spatula. Every few minutes, whisk the chocolate to make sure it's completely melted. Set it momentarily over a double boiler with simmering water if all of the chocolate doesn't melt and the chocolate is cold.)

Pour the filling into the chilled pie crust and allow it to set for at least one hour. At room temperature, serve the tart. Refrigerate any leftovers for up to a week in an airtight container.

To make a dry rub for meat, grind up lavender and other herbs like rosemary and thyme and mix them together. Crispy Marjoram Potatoes (page 89) are a great place to use it, along with the marjoram. Try making lavender ice cream by steeping lavender blossoms in milk.

Puff Pastry with Lovage and Blackberries

The aromatic seeds of lovage, a herb commonly employed in savoury dishes, can also be used in sweet treats. Spicy foods, such as the peaches in this crisp, go particularly well with them. Baked

Simple and quick to make, fruit crisps are a great dessert option. The lovage seeds and peaches and blackberries in this dessert make it ideal for serving in the waning days of summer. Make a side of ice cream or whipped cream and serve the crisp with that on the side. If you have any leftovers, store them in the refrigerator or at room temperature carefully wrapped in parchment paper.

4 to 6 people can be fed with this dish.

Filling

Cut the peaches into large bits and put them in a large pot.

- Blackberries, 11.2 pounds
- 1 cup of sugar
- Topping

Whole wheat pastry flour: • 14 cup

- 12 cup oats, rolled

Sugar, brown, 12 cup

- 14 cup pecans finely chopped
- 112 tsp. cinnamon ground
- 1 tsp. lovage seeds, finely ground

Nutmeg freshly grated to taste, 14 teaspoon

Salt, about a quarter-teaspoon

At least 6 tbsp unsalted butter in the fridge

Pre-heat the oven to 350°F

Toss the fruit with the sugar in a large bowl. Prepare a baking dish by pouring in the mixture.

You may make the topping by combining all of the dry ingredients (flour through salt) with the wet ingredients (oatmeal through brown sugar) in a bowl. Assemble the ingredients into a coarse crumb and large chunks with your fingertips. Once the butter has been incorporated and the topping has come together, use a spatula to distribute it over the fruit.

Bake for 40 to 45 minutes, rotating the pan halfway through baking, until the crisp is golden brown and the fluids are bubbling up the sides.

Lovage seeds are an excellent spice to keep on hand for garden recipes. Roasting and grilling foods can benefit from the addition of ground cloves. In most recipes, lovage can be used in place of fennel seeds.

Icing on the Blackberry, Buttermilk

Using low-fat buttermilk and minimal sugar, this blackberry buttermilk ice cream is practically guilt-free. Clean city-picked blackberries well before using (see Blackberry Jam, page 120). Thierry, my chef friend, taught me years ago how to regulate the freezing temperature of ice cream. I've never figured out how he does it, but his sorbets are to die for. Booze makes the combination feel less "icy" by raising the freezing point and thereby reducing its harshness. It's a good idea to keep this in your wallet.

- One pint of beer
- Blackberries, 12 pound (about 2 cups)

16 ounces of honey

Low-fat buttermilk: • 1 cup

At least one tbsp.

For 30 minutes on your counter, combine the blackberries and sugar in a bowl. When the fruit is ripe, combine it with the buttermilk and vodka in a blender until smooth. To remove the seeds and hairs from the blackberries, pour the mixture through a fine mesh sieve.

Frozen until creamy and solidified, as directed by the manufacturer in an ice cream machine, using a spatula to scrape down the edges as needed. If you plan on serving ice cream at a later date, keep it in an airtight container in the freezer.

Try the crisp or blackberry jam for more blackberry recipe ideas from the garden.

Ice with Lemon Verbena Flavors

In the sweltering heat of summer, nothing beats an icy treat or beverage. Midsummer is the ideal time of year for lemon verbena since it thrives in the heat. Once clipped, it will soon regrow and be quite prolific. This is a simple recipe that can be used with a variety of herbs, making it versatile. In essence, it's a frozen wine-infused simple syrup. Every 15 minutes or so, you must rake the ice crystals through the mixture to generate icy granita. There is no smoothness to the sorbet-like dessert that develops from this method. The granita can also be used in beverages. Add some to a cocktail glass with gin and a splash of soda for a nighttime drink. A garnish of fresh lemon verbena leaves is a nice touch.

4 to 6 people can be fed with this dish.

• 2 cups of water

Sugar, 2 cups, 1 teaspoon

Lemon verbena leaves ranging from 20 to 30

For the sauvignon blanc: • 1 cup of light, crisp white wine

At least one tablespoon of lemon juice

Bring the water, sugar, and lemon verbena leaves to a boil in a medium saucepan. Remove the pan from the heat, add the sugar, and allow the lemon verbena steep for a few minutes. Make sure the lemon verbena flavour is prominent after the water is cooled down. Bring to a boil and continue to steep until desired flavour is achieved. Pour the mixture into a shallow baking dish and let it sit until the flavours are just right before adding the wine. Frozen is the only option. To see if the liquid has partially frozen, check back in 20 minutes. Return to the freezer after removing any ice crystals with a fork. Repeat in 15 minutes. Once the entire mixture is flaky and frozen, stop stirring and let it sit for another 30 minutes or more.

Lemon verbena is a frequent herb in teas, but it's also great when steeped on its own with a little honey. Its leaves can be used to make ice cream or custard by steeping them in cream. Lamb and other gamey meats go well with this herb. Marinate lamb chops or steaks with chopped leaves. In some recipes, lemon zest can be substituted with lemon verbena.

Chapter Seven

CANNING FOR THE BATHROOM

Water-bath canning is explained in detail here. There are a few choices, but they are all effective. Set up your jars and workspace in advance so that you can get into a routine. In addition, pay attention to the processing times specified in each recipe.

The Jars Need to be Cleaned

Rinse the jars and lids in hot soapy water, then place them on a drying rack or dish towel to dry completely.

Setting Up the Jars

You do not need to sanitise glass jars and lids before using them in boiling water baths or pressure canners if you plan to process your food for longer than 10 minutes. Jars must be sterilised before filling if the processing time is shorter than 10 minutes. Do this by bringing the water in the jars to a simmer in a canning kettle with the lid on and the jars inside. To keep them fresh, keep the jars in water. As an alternative, I always warm up jars that have just been washed in a 225°F oven until they are ready to be used. The USDA does not endorse this, but since I'm still here, I'll give it to you anyhow.

Intake of Liquid

It's all about the labels.

Label each jar with the date and the contents after it has cooled. Jars that have been properly sealed should be kept in a cool, dark location, such as a cupboard. However, I've let canned items sit for several months past the recommended expiration date with no ill effects.

In the Details

Apple Butter with Rose Hip Butter

These rose fruits, which are best picked in the middle of summer, are one of my all-time favourite foraging treats. Rose hips are rather fibrous, so they require a good bit of preparation before they can be used in recipes. It can take a long time and a lot of attention to prepare fruit butters properly. It's worth the time and effort to make this butter, which has a delicate but distinct rose scent and transforms apple butter into something very special.

- Five half-pint jars are produced.

At least 2 pounds of rhubarb

11.5 pounds of tart apples, cleaned and sliced into 1-inch chunks •

• 3 cups of sugar.

• Juice of 1 lemon, reserved halves

Rinse the rose hips and remove the stems and ends. Fill a big pot halfway with water, then add the rose hips. Bring water to a boil, then simmer for 30 to 45 minutes until the vegetables are tender. Retain the pulp from the rose hips after they've been put through a food mill. A few passes may be necessary to remove all of the fruit's peel, seeds, and hairs. Remove any seeds from the rose hips by squeezing them through a fine mesh strainer. This will collect any stray hairs or seeds that may have gotten loose.

Add enough water to cover the apples in a stockpot. Bring to a simmer over medium-high heat. You're ready to mash the fruit when it's soft enough to do so with a spoon.

Make a batch at a time by placing half of the apples in the blender and pulverising. Back into the pot with a fine mesh strainer, add the apple purée. Return the liquid to medium heat and add the rose hip purée, sugar, and lemon juice and half.

Cook at a low to medium heat, constantly stirring to prevent burning of the fruit butter. Reduce the heat if it's getting too hot and burning the bottom of the pot. When a small amount of butter is placed on a cool dish, no liquid separates from the solid to form a ring around it, the butter is done. For this, you'll need at least an hour and a half.

Remove the lemon halves from the fruit butter once it has reached the desired consistency. Fill glass jars with butter and seal them. It can be kept for several weeks in the refrigerator.

Cooking down the rose hips and sweetening them all on their own makes the rosy flavour more prominent. There are many ways to include rose hip purée into your culinary repertoire, from pairing it with cheese to using it in fruit pies.

Capers of Nasturtium

This plant's entire life cycle can be consumed, from the roots to its flowers to its seeds. It looks like a little nutmeg, with somewhat wrinkled and crevice-covered skins when the seeds are young. When the seeds are the size of a pea, remove them from the plant. As with capers, young nasturtium seeds can be brined or pickled with vinegar. Add a pickled crunch to pastas and salads. The refrigerator is a great place to keep both brined and pickled seeds. Pickled seeds should be used within three weeks of being made; after that, they begin to degrade and become mushy. The seeds grow in cycles, thus these are manufactured in tiny quantities like authentic capers.

One-half cup

Nasturtium seeds, 12 cup

A tablespoon of ground coriander

- 1 tsp. ground mustard
- 3 cloves, whole

salt, about a half tsp.

Rice wine vinegar, about a half-cup

A quarter-cup sweetener

Gather all of the ingredients for the nasturtiums, coriander, and mustard seeds in a pint-sized jar and store them in a cool area. In a small saucepan, combine the rice wine vinegar and sugar and bring to a boil over high heat. Pour the vinegar into the jar while it's still hot. Leave at room temperature for a few minutes before serving. Refrigerate after securing the jar's cover. Let the "capers" ferment for at least a day before eating.

Spices can be varied in the pickling mixture if desired. Garlic, red chilli flakes, or pieces of fresh gingerroot are all good options.

Jam made with Blackberry Berries

In August, blackberries are in abundance, so it's a good idea to carry a bowl in your car so you can stop and pick them whenever the need strikes. To make the most of roadside blackberries, soak them for a few minutes first. Pour them into a large bowl of ice-cold water and gently whisk them around. The bugs and hairs will be released as well. Before draining the berries entirely, remove the top layer of debris. You can stock your cupboard and extend the season by preserving berries. If you want to produce a syrup instead of jam, you can simmer it down for a shorter period of time.

It yields four half-pint jars

At least 2 pounds of freshly-picked blackberries

• 3 cups of sugar.

Lemons sliced in half are included in this package.

Large saucepan: Add the berries and sugar and bring to a boil. Add both halves of the lemon to the pot and squeeze off the juice. Natural pectin is added to your jam to help it set, so this is a good thing to do.

Set on a medium-low flame. Cook for about 20 minutes, or until the berries begin to lose their juice and begin to break down. Remove from the heat, cover, and store in the refrigerator for at least one night.

Put a plate in the freezer in the morning. You'll use this to see if your jam is all the way set.

Break down the berries by simmering them in a pot over medium-low heat for about 20 minutes. The lemon halves and any seeds should be thrown away. Using a blender, mix the blackberries until they are a smooth pulp. A fine mesh strainer should be placed over the pot of jam to remove any seeds. Cook the jam over a medium-low heat, stirring frequently, until it reaches the desired consistency. Place a tablespoon of your jam on a cooled dish to see if it has set. Jam should wrinkle when pressed gently with a finger, but the fruit spoon should remain whole. Cooking time ranges from 30 to 40 minutes on average.. You can use less time and remove from heat when the purée becomes a loose sauce if you'd want to produce blackberry syrup.) Pour the jam into jars and process in a hot water bath for 5 minutes after it's done cooking (see Water-Bath Canning 101 on page 116).

If you want to store berries in your freezer, lay them out in one layer on a sheet pan and put them in the freezer one by one. Stock up on frozen fruit for winter smoothies and pies in resealable plastic bags.

Chapter Eight

Syrup with Herbs

Sugar and water make up the simple syrup. You can add everything from fresh herbs or flowers to dried spices or teas to simple syrups for infusions. The Rosy Strawberries with Buttermilk Cake on page 106 is a great example of how simple syrups may be used as a flavouring agent for fresh fruit or as a glaze for cakes. They're a subtle method to give a little bit of flavour without going overboard. Take your pick of any herb. Adding a few drops of lavender essential oil to a vanilla or chocolate cake will enhance the flavour. Fresh berries and anise hyssop simple syrup are a match made in heaven. To make a delicately flavoured syrup to drizzle over pancakes or yoghurt, gather rose hips from the wild and cook them down. Frozen syrup granita makes for a simple after-school snack or after-dinner treat!

Makes one cup

• 1 cup of sugar

approximately one-half cup of liquid

Spices, herbs, and other botanicals: • 3 tablespoons

The ingredients should be mixed together and heated in a small saucepan. Afterwards, remove it from the heat and allow it to soak for a few minutes with the herbs. After 15 minutes, take a taste and see if it's to your satisfaction. Strain the syrup and use it as directed if the syrup contains solids. The syrup can be kept in the fridge for several weeks. If the flavour isn't strong enough, keep steeping the herbs until you're happy. For a stronger infusion, drain the utilised herbs and re-heat the infused mixture with new herbs, using the same procedure each time.

Garden Tisanes (page 134) and herbal sun teas can be made with extra herbs and flowers. Sugar or salt can also be used to crush herbs for garnish or flavouring.

Cordial made with chamomile

Sweetened syrups infused with herbs, spices, or plants are known as cordials. Making them is a breeze, and the possibilities for taste combinations are endless. For a grown-up non-alcoholic "cocktail," cordials are the right solution. Use fresh or dried chamomile flowers for this syrup.

Drinking chamomile infusions in the heat of summer is a pleasant way to enjoy the herb's medical benefits (as well as its calming effect). Crush some ice and add some syrup to a bottle of fizzy water before serving. If you don't want the floral flavour to be overpowered by cognac, add a splash. A basic yellow or buttermilk cake drizzled with this syrup is also a great way to enjoy it.

This recipe yields roughly two cups.

1 teaspoon dried lavender flowers (or 3 teaspoons fresh lavender petals)

flowers of chamomile

Boiling water for 2 cups

- 14 cup granulated honey

- 2 cups of slushy water

Slices of cucumber as a finishing touch

This includes bourbon and tequila (optional)

Chamomile blossoms can be steeped in tea bags or strainers made of fine mesh. Use a fine mesh strainer to keep the chamomile seeds from escaping and floating in your syrup. Steep in the hot water for about 20 minutes, or until the liquid becomes yellow and smells strongly of thyme. Press any remaining liquid out of the muslin bag and discard the solids, then flush the bag. Take a small amount of honey and mix it in with the rest of the ingredients. Refrigerate for at least one hour before serving.

Add crushed ice to a glass once the syrup has cooled. Pour roughly half a cup of the chamomile cordial into each serving and top with half a cup of seltzer water. Add a tiny slice of cucumber as a finishing touch. If you'd like, serve with a splash of cognac on the side.

Refrigerate the cordial after making it, and it will keep for a few weeks.

Chamomile can be used for lovage seeds in the topping of the Blackberry Peach Crisp with Lovage (page 112). Chamomile heads can also be used to produce a calming tea by drying them.

In order to maintain a vacuum in cooling jars, all canned items will require headspace. All jams and jellies should have a 14-inch headspace, while entire fruits should have a 12-inch headspace. When using entire fruits, tap the jar on the counter or place a wooden chopstick or skewer into the jar and gently mix the fruit to dislodge air bubbles. Canning jar rings should not be overtightened while putting lids and rings on them. Just tighten the rings to the point where they feel snug. Overtightening the jars prevents air from escaping, which is an essential part of canning.

The Canning Pot is being heated.

Half-fill your canning pan with water and bring it to a gentle boil. Keep the liquid at a low simmer until you're ready to use it.

Preparation for canning

Place the prepared jars of food in the canner on the rack if you're using a canning pot. To ensure proper water circulation for sealing, do not stack. Add enough water to cover the jars by an inch or more to the canning kettle. Return the saucepan to a boil, then remove the lid. The canning process begins when the water in the canning pot is brought back to a rolling boil. Keep an eye on your pot and a timer nearby as this can take up to 15 minutes. In small batches, you may also use a stockpot by covering the bottom with a dish towel and stacking your jars on top. This prevents the jars from banging against the pot's bottom or falling over. Although the USDA does not advocate this method of canning, I've seen farmers and European country folk utilise it, and I've adopted their laissez-faire approach.

Taking Away the Sealed Jars

When the processing time is up, remove the jars from the canner with a jar lifter or a pair of kitchen tongs. After the canning kettle is brought back to a boil, the processing period will begin.) Refrigerate the jars for at least an hour on a folded towel. Make sure you don't create an artificial seal by pressing down on the tops.

The Art of Sealing Glass Jars

As soon as you hear the sound of can tops popping, you know the seal is strong. Once the jars have cooled, remove the outer ring and lift the jar with the lid only to ensure a proper seal. If it doesn't fall apart, you've done a good job canning your food. You can reprocess in the water bath within twenty-four hours if the seal is damaged or loose. Make sure you use a fresh lid and inspect the jar rim for cracks or nicks. Alternatively, you can store the jar in the refrigerator and utilise it within three weeks of opening it.

Do-It-Yourself Flower Bed

Making your own lip balm or tea is a simple but effective way to bring the garden into your daily routine. It's a terrific way to improve your creative thinking skills. I've frequently sat in my garden and contemplated what I could make from the little farm I've grown as I looked around. I'm a sucker for everything homemade, and my cabinets are stocked with anything from flavoured sugars and salts to homemade crackers and jams.

My first thought is, "I can do that," when I see something I like that appears to be readily constructed. Particularly those containing no more than five ingredients. The garden is a great source of inspiration for DIY projects.

Looking at my plants a few years ago, I was thinking about what I could do with them. Aside from the fact that I enjoy looking at my scented geraniums, I prefer to raise things that produce in numerous ways. Ritzy, a friend and neighbour of mine, was a big fan of organic cosmetic products and environmental sustainability. Every time I visited mom, I'd go prowling around the shelves and squirt some cream or apply some oil on my skin. Something I'd never spend money on was opulent and opulent. My desire to manufacture my own items was sparked by my mother's encouragement and the strength of my own plants. Facial toner was my first step. The use of a toner may appear to be needless to some.

Astringent characteristics (which are nice when you're working out in the sun and sweating all day) and it smells beautiful. Toner is not something I use. What's the harm in making a little batch of something exceptional if I have all the components at my disposal? Even men can benefit from a little bit of toner, so it's not just for women. Men, too, can benefit from a daily application of an astringent.

Your garden's ripe and ready-to-harvest produce can inspire this and many other garden ideas. Trimming a plant when there is no evident use for what I harvest is common for me. When that happens, I stop preparing dinner and go to my cupboards to see if there's a way to store or use what I've got. Making your own beauty products is a simple and thoughtful hostess gift. You can also produce your own teas, rubs, and flavoured salts by drying your herbs. These are all great reminders that the summer sun will return when there are no plants to be found in the winter.

Some of my favourite DIY garden projects are included here.

Chapter Nine

Cosmetic Toner

APOTHECARY OF HERBAL MEDICINE

My mother used to keep a giant bottle of witch hazel astringent in our bathroom cabinet when I was a child. In order to stay cool during the summer, my sister and I would soak cotton balls in water and then rub them against our skin. My mom probably kept it around because of its ability to tone and tighten the skin. I still enjoy the scent of witch hazel to this day. Adapted from Rosemary Gladstar's Herbal Recipes for Vibrant Health, this toner cleans and tightens pores while also removing excess oil from the face. Because vinegar serves as a preservative in this toner, it can be stored for a long time without losing its effectiveness. Although the toner does have a mild vinegar scent, it is not overpowering and does not linger on the skin. The toning properties of witch hazel are utilised in equal measure. As a bonus, I'm including my favourite herb combination.

The herbs may be changed, but it's up to you. One need is that your herbs must always be completely soaked in vinegar after they are introduced.

Floral and mint Toner

- 10 petals of the rose geranium

Ten chamomile heads are included.

- 6 sprigs of lemon balm
- 6 mint fronds

One cup of apple cider vinegar made using organic apples

- 1 14 cups witch hazel berries

Using hot, soapy water, rinse and dry the jar. Add the herbs and flowers to the jar by tearing and squeezing them. Pour the vinegar over the flowers and herbs when it is hot but not boiling. Keep it in a dark, cool place for 2 to 3 weeks before using. The herbs should always be immersed.

Strain out the herbs after a few weeks have elapsed. The witch hazel should be incorporated into the mixture by sprinkling it in. Toner can be stored in a small glass container and used to freshly cleaned skin every day.

infused oils

Oil is used as a carrier for the plant's own oil and aroma in infused oils, essential oils, and solar-infused oils. Infusions prepared with olive oil are the most common. When utilised on their own, infused oils can be used for everything from moisturising the skin to serving as a flavouring ingredient in food (no joke). Temperature and light can have a negative effect on the durability of infused oils, so keep them in a dark, cold place. Properly preserved, they will last for weeks, if not years. Keep your jars and utensils totally dry before bottling, and use dry herbs instead of fresh ones.

Chapter Ten

HERB DRYING

It's a great method to extend your crop, and it's a fun activity to do in your spare time. Herbs are known for their rapid growth. Fast-growing plants and hectic schedules make it difficult for many home gardeners to harvest fresh herbs in time. Active trimming and stimulation of new growth is also beneficial to these plants. I've seen herbs bloom when they should be trimmed down and utilised in a dish. It's time to try herb drying if your herbs are growing too fast for you to use them in your cooking.

To preserve fresh herbs, keep them in a warm, dry location. Yeast, bacteria, and mould can harm herb-saving initiatives if there is too much moisture present during the drying process. Cut herbs almost all the way to the root, but leave a few green leaves and some room for them to grow back. What to Grow, For Real: Chapter 3, What to Grow, For Real: Chapter 3, What to Grow, For Real: Using a tray or a hanging method, herbs can be dried. Dry herbs by tying the stems together and hanging them from a hook in the ceiling. To dry herbs in a tray, set the cuttings on a parchment-lined baking sheet and rotate them every few hours or so to prevent moisture from building up beneath the leaves. Generally speaking, it takes four to six days for most herbs to dry out. When they disintegrate readily when touched, they are completely dry.

Making infused oil can be accomplished in one of two ways. One option is a simple one that can be completed in a single day. Using low heat on the stove or oven, herbs are heated until they release their essential oils and scents into the carrier oil. Alternatively, you can use the light and heat of the sun to infuse your herbs, which will gradually warm them and aid release their essential oils. In the event that you are able to devote the necessary time and resources, you should choose for sun infusion. The ideal infusions are those that are lengthy, gradual, and low-maintenance.

Make sure you start with clean herbs for all infusions. Rinse your herbs and flowers in a bowl of cool water if they have soil or dust on them. In order to eliminate some of the moisture, place a towel between two layers of towels and press them together to dry. Make sure to shift the leaves around and make sure they aren't overlapping as this can take a long time.

When herbs are dried, they can be fragile and easily dispersed. If I want to ensure that I get all of the dry leaves, seeds or flowers, I will typically place the herbs in a large paper bag while still holding the connected stems. I either shake the dried leaves into the bag or carefully pull the entire stem through my fist to remove them, depending on how much time I have to spend. This method ensures that you're catching all of the leaves or seeds rather than scattering them throughout the house! The stems should be completely free of all the leaves, so pour them onto a clean counter or sheet pan. Separate the plant leaves from any stems or debris before using. Using a gentle breeze, you may blow on a small pile of leaves and they will sort themselves—leaves moving away from the "breeze," as it were. Clean the leaves and place them in a glass jar in your spice cabinet. You can use a dough scraper or a spoon to achieve this (which should be cool, dry, and far from any heat sources).

Of course, some herbs dry out better than others. Listed here is a small list of herbs that are easy to grow and great pantry fillers:.

Citrus Bergamot

The herb Lemon Verbena

- Marjoram

- Mint

- Rosemary
- Sage
- Thyme
- Infusion on the Stovetop

olive oil, about a cup

As many as two handfuls of herbs or flowers, if possible

Using a small saucepan, warm the olive oil and herbs. For at least two hours and up to eight, gently whisk the mixture. Steeping an oil is complete when the aroma is unmistakable. In order to extract all of the plant's essential oil, use a fine-mesh strainer to remove all leaves and branches. If you'd like an even stronger aroma, repeat the process with already-infused oil.

Until you're ready to use the oil, keep it covered in a dark, cool cupboard.

Fusion of the sun's energy

1 cup of extra virgin olive oil

2 sprigs of flowers or herbs

In a quart-sized glass jar, combine the oil with the herbs or flowers. Make sure the oil covers all the plant stuff. The jar should be covered and placed in the sun to steep for at least two weeks. During the day, be sure to rotate it around so that it's always in the sun.

To remove any remaining leaves and branches, use a fine mesh strainer and press against them to extract all the plant oils. If you'd like an even stronger aroma, repeat the process with already-infused oil.

Lip Balm is

The Quillisascut Farm School in Eastern Washington had me thinking about all the wonderful things we could do with herbs while I was there in the spring of last year. Lora Lea stepped away from the table in the middle of a conversation and returned with a large jug of green oil. THyme-infused oil was a delectable treat. We started making lip balm right away, and I was fascinated. Using infused oil and beeswax turned out to be quite simple, despite my previous fears. Natural food stores and co-ops are a good source of beeswax. Cuticle and elbow salve can be quickly made using this method. You may even want to eat it, but don't. It smells so nice.

Lip Balm with Thyme

• 2 large sprigs of thyme, washed thoroughly

olive oil, about a cup

Two ounces of grated beeswax

Olive oil and herbs can be warmed in a small pot over low heat. Stirring occasionally, let steep for a few hours. Because of the thyme leaves, the oil will become green. Strain off the leaves and stems using a fine mesh strainer.

Put the oil back on a low heat and whisk in the beeswax until it has melted. Remove the pan from the heat and use an electric mixer to combine the ingredients. This makes the salve super-creamy and fluffier.

Put it in small jars or tins when it has turned a lighter shade of green and has grown in volume. Allow to cool before tightly sealing the container.

Soothing Lotion

Lip balms and salves are very similar products, with the only difference being their consistency. Beeswax is needed in greater quantities in lip balms to ensure that they stay cohesive. Skin balms can retain some of their gentler qualities after being applied. It's possible to utilise salves for both hydrating and therapeutic purposes. Lavender oil can be applied topically to stings, bites, and scrapes to relieve itching and irritation. Invigorating and revitalising, mint salve is a great after-workout pick-me-up. Try any flower or herb you choose, but don't mix herbs and flowers in one infusion—keep it simple. Separate them if you want to combine two infusions.

If you save each infusion for a specific smell, you'll have more creative freedom.

Oil of Oregano

a gramme of beeswax

Infused oil: 12 c.

The salve will absorb the flavours of the other foods in the kitchen if the beeswax and infused oil are not combined in a small pot that is used solely for this purpose. Afterwards, transfer the mixture to small containers and seal them with lids or bandages.

Pantry of herbs

SALTS FROM HERBS

When I was a kid, I had an abundance of lovage seeds in one of my gardens a few years ago. I went down there late one summer day and discovered that the entire plant had gone to seed. All the stems were chopped off, and the seed-filled flower heads were taken home where they were dried out on racks. For the rest of the year, I had enough of lovage seeds in my spice cabinet thanks to that small detour. In fact, I still have some! I created some savoury salt with the leftover seeds, and my pals have been clamouring for it. Whether it's the powerful and distinctive aroma or its versatility, this salt rub is a definite winner in my book. I'm not sure what it is, but this salt rub is a definite winner in my book.

Herb salts are fantastic since they may be used in so many different ways. You can use them for a variety of purposes, including seasoning meat, dressing salads, and sprinkling grains. A wide variety of salts can be used to make salt blends. I prefer kosher salt because it isn't as mineral-tasting as some sea salts, and it isn't as coarse as some sea salts. So that the seeds are completely mixed with the salt, I prefer to pound them in a mortar and pestle. Salt and herbs or flowers can simply be tossed together. In terms of food preservation, it's worth noting that salt can help. To prevent spoiling, salt can be used to remove moisture from herbs, which is a risk factor for mould.

Here are a few garden-inspired ideas to get you started; don't be afraid to try something new.

Sulfuric Acid (from Flowers)

The maturation of numerous herbs occurs at the same time, thus they will bloom at the same time as well. Cutting back flowering herbs may be necessary, but you may not always have a use for them. Whenever I don't have time to cook with them, I use them in a herbal salt. Chive and thyme flowers complement each other nicely in terms of flavour, so they make excellent dinner party guests. Check the flavour after a few days of salting the chive blossoms because they have a powerful onion flavour.

Amount of chive blossoms:

- 3 tbsp. dried thyme flower

Salt (kosher): one and a half cups

Remove the flowers' stems and arrange them in a basin. Stir in the salt until it is well-combined. Salt to the point where it is at least equal to the amount of blooms. If you don't like the flavour, you can always add a little more salt to balance it out.

LOVAGE SALT:

As lovage seeds are so flavorful, this is a terrific way to get them into your diet. If you want to get the most out of them, smash them with a mortar and pestle first.

Lovage seed (dried): three tablespoons

Kosher salt: 1 cup

Crush and grind lovage seeds until they are at least a third of their original size with a mortar and pestle. Crush some of the salt in the mortar while you combine it with the other half. Stir in the rest of the salt using a rubber spatula to make sure it's all incorporated. When pressing seeds into a mortar, use a rubber spatula to remove any oils from the seeds. Store in a cold, dark cupboard until ready to use in a glass jar or small container with a tight-fitting lid.

The Tisanes Garden

Another word for herbal tea is tisane. It's smart to create teas if you've got a little urban garden so that you can get a taste of your garden all year round! Making a tisane and adding honey to it is one of my go-to remedies for sick plants or leaves that are starting to turn. Herbs are used for a variety of purposes, some of which are therapeutic. To prepare a tisane at home, I often use whatever ingredients I have on hand and am in the mood for. Stomach-soothing herbs like mint and anise hyssop include these. Mint is a stimulant in and of itself. Chamomile has a relaxing effect.

It is possible to make tisanes out of either fresh or dried herbs. The strength of dried leaves is higher. For every cup of water, add 3 tablespoons of fresh herbs or flowers, or 1 tablespoon of dried herbs.

When you dry your own herbs, you can make a wide variety of tea blends at home. Alternatively, you can store individual dried plants and mix a custom blend to your specifications. All of my herbs are stored separately in glass jars, and I only use a small amount at a time. Garden tisanes can be made with the following combinations:

Hyssop and mint are a match made in heaven.

Mint, Lemon Balm, and Anise Hyssop

Lavender with Chamomile

Mint, Lovage, and Chamomile

Combination of Lavender, Mint, and Geranium

Lemon verbena with lavender

Rose geranium paired with lemon verbena

Infused Spirits with Herbs

Another way to use up some of the herbs and spices you've harvested from your garden is to infuse whiskey with them. Spirits' high alcohol concentration serves as a preservative, reducing the risk of contamination. Most spirits can be infused, but vodka, gin, and light rum are the finest because they are clear and pure. Herbal-infused liqueurs are wonderful holiday presents. During the summer months, stock up on supplies; your friends will thank you for it come winter.

Infusing your spirits with fruit and herbs is also an option. Oxbow Farms' founders, Luke and Sarah, are continuously infusing or combining something with their garden glut, which I admire much. They brewed rum with plums and chamomile last year since their plum tree yielded just too much fruit to eat fresh. They drank the rum and baked an upside-down cake with the soaking fruit.

Add the herbs to a glass jar and mash the leaves with the handle of a wooden spoon to release the oils. Just enough alcohol to barely cover them. Store in a cool, dark cupboard with a tight-fitting cap. It is important to shake spirit infusions a couple times a day. Try it for yourself after three days to determine if the flavour is right or if it needs more time to settle in. In general, it takes five to seven days for a flavour to develop, although the length of time depends entirely on you.

Strain the herbs and return the infused spirits to a container that can be sealed if the flavour is just right for you. Refrigerate until ready to use and keep in a cool, dark place

Try these combinations of herbs and spirits:

gin with anise hyssop

Lovage and Gin

Mint and gin

Chamomile and rum

Vodka and basil in a cocktail

Lemon verbena and bourbon

Chapter Eleven

SEE AND FEEL THE WORLD AROUND YOU

Plant Labels with a Twist

I'm not sure why people spend money on stuff they could manufacture at home, when they could do it themselves. As long as you're not growing on a huge scale and need to buy labels in bulk, plant labels fall into this category. I love my garden to seem uniform, so I spend some time on the design and feel of my plant labels. Starts often arrive with labels.

Labels for Seed Starting

When it comes to seed beginning, having clearly labelled plants is critical. It's nearly tough to identify little plants with only a few leaves. It takes a long time and a lot of repetition to get good at it. It is common to start seeds in big seed trays covered by plastic sheets. For this reason, labels must be both tiny enough not to obstruct the cover and large enough to include the information you want to include on them. It's important to select a material that won't degrade quickly, since you'll be watering it frequently. I found this out the hard way when I tried to make labels from strips of heavy cardstock paper the first year. It's surprising that no one has developed a labelling system specifically for home gardeners. I'm happy to report that after years of trial and error, I've come up with a simple, inexpensive, and useful solution.

Bamboo skewers and clear tape are a must. Each label is made by cutting a skewer into four-inch pieces. Cut the tape to a length that's about the same. Use masking tape to make an inverted flag by placing one end of the short bamboo skewer directly on top of another end of the tape and then wrapping the tape around it. You may now write on both sides of the tape with a ballpoint pen because the tape has adhered to itself. In addition to the seed's name and estimated maturity date, I usually include (45 days, 65 days, and so on).

The Plant Labels were gathered.

Rocks and river stones can be used as plant markers in an urban garden. When you're out for a walk or near a mountain stream, keep an eye out. Because containers don't appreciate extra weight, it's best to keep everything as light as possible. A permanent marker and a piece of paper can be used to write directly on the rocks. You'll need to either rewrite the label every few months or cover it with a quick coat of clear gloss paint because the writing will fade over time in the sun.

Vintage Cutlery and Cutlery Sets

When my friend Marcus was out "junking" years ago, he picked up some mismatched silverware for me. Large soup spoons and long butter knives with scrolls and hobnails were given to me by him. However, the metal was so worn that it generated a peculiar metallic reaction in my mouth; I would never use them to eat. I put them in the back of my silver drawer and completely forgot about them.

In the future, I discovered a blog post featuring tchotchkes made out of exactly identical type of cutlery. For an outdoor plant label, I decided to use the spoons' charming faces as a starting point for my own design. I tried it out and was blown away by the results. To make these labels, all you need is some white glue and some old cutlery. Glue for decoupage projects is something I always keep on hand, even if there are more specialised glues on the market. In the end, I never looked into anything more "professional" because it worked for me the first time. In the bowl or handle, cut off a piece of plain white paper that is long enough to fit along the handle or inside the spoon. Using a fine-tipped pen or marker, write down the plant's name on this label. Let the white glue dry completely before attaching the label on the handle or spoon bowl. Mix two parts white glue with one part water to make a glue wash. Ideally, it should be light and sticky. Brush over the label with a little paintbrush, being sure to cover it thoroughly but lightly, to prevent any lines from appearing. Apply a second application when the first one has dried. Reapply a third and final coat of paint. There are a few things you can do if you want your labels to support our initiative.

Spray a clear UV- and water-resistant substance over the top to ensure that it lasts a long time. Housewares and hardware businesses carry these. Using the bowl of a spoon as a potting label, insert the handle of the cutlery into the potting soil once it is completely dry.

Labels You Can Make and Bake

In order to do this project, you'll need to gather some supplies, which is both exciting and terrifying. No purchase rule is broken, but it is worth it. Are you familiar with Shrinky Dinks? They were one of my favourite cartoon characters when I was younger. Afterwards, I'd bake them and watch as they turned into small plastic figurines. While attending a craft fair a few years ago, I saw a seller selling Shrinky Dink earrings. I took her idea and applied it to plant tags, and the results were stunning. Sheets of Shrinky Dink can be acquired in most local toy stores or online, depending on your location. The only secret is to make the label large enough so that the print is legible. Normally, I cut a five-by-two-inch section of plastic for a plant label. You'll get a sign that's about a two by one inch after baking this. Black ink on a white background appeals to me, but you can be more imaginative and use colour. Use a thin, pointed marker or coloured pencil for this project, just like you did for the silverware labels, to ensure exact lettering. You can also cut and bake clear squares, and then write the plant name with a pencil after baking them. In the long run, you can remove and reapply the labels.

In order to properly place the label on the plant container, you must first plan out your strategy. There is no need to apply the label to the ground before planting. Make a small hole in the top of your label before baking so that you can tie it to the base of your plant with string, thread, or ribbon. Another option is to punch a small hole straight across from one another on each side of the label (with the help of a small hole punch). Unfold two paper clips and the wire through the hole on both sides of the label, after baking the label. In order to keep the label in place, penetrate the earth with this tent post.

The Containers Are Spray-Painted

Plastic containers irritate me because of their appearance. For the price, they're fantastic to have, but they're not particularly attractive because of that. When I use a plastic pot, I take up a can of spray paint and give it a new look. Spray paints are available in a wide variety of hues, so you may use them to enhance the aesthetics of your outdoor environment. If you like a more subdued look, you can use any colour you like—blues, yellows, and reds are all good options.

Work outside in a well-ventilated area (on a quiet day), far from buildings or cars, to paint your pot. You don't want to paint your neighbor's car by accident with spray paint because it disperses so swiftly in the air. Protect the ground or grass you're working on by laying down three times as much newspaper as the pot. It's best to keep the can six inches away from the pot and move it slowly across its surface. I use my left hand to turn the container while I spray with my right. Only a few inches down from the pot's rim should be sprayed. More soil will be added to the pot to complete the interior. When spraying, keep the can at least a few inches away from the surface you're painting to avoid paint drip marks. This isn't endearing at all. Let the pot dry thoroughly between coats. To dry entirely, it takes around fifteen minutes. Paint three coats on the surface.

CPSIA information can be obtained
at www.ICGtesting.com
Printed in the USA
LVHW061208190722
723853LV00014B/562

9 781804 768778